Beginners Guide To CBD HEMP OIL

What you need to know

DISCLAIMER

The information contained in and its components, is meant to serve as a comprehensive collection of strategies that the author of this eBook has done research about. Summaries, strategies, tips and tricks are only recommendations by the author, and reading this eBook will not guarantee that one's results will exactly mirror the author's results.

The author of this Ebook has made all reasonable efforts to provide current and accurate information for the readers of this eBook. The author and its associates will not be held liable for any unintentional errors or omissions that may be found.

The material in the Ebook may include information by third parties. Third party materials comprise of opinions expressed by their owners. As such, the author of this eBook does not assume responsibility or liability for any third party material or opinions. The publication of third party material does not constitute the author's guarantee of any information, products, services, or opinions contained within third party material. Use of third party material does not guarantee that your results will mirror our results. Publication of such third party material is simply a recommendation and expression of the author's own opinion of that material.

Whether because of the progression of the Internet, or the unforeseen changes in company policy and editorial submission guidelines, what is stated as fact at the time of this writing may become outdated or inapplicable later.

TABLE OF CONTENT

HEMP OIL

Hemp oil comes from the hemp seed and it has been traditionally used in lubricants, paint, ink manufacture, fuel and plastic products. It is also used in the production of skin care products, natural soaps, shampoos and detergents. In recent years, hemp seed oil has been recognized as natures most balanced oil for human nutrition with the perfect three to one Omega three to Omega six ratio required by the human body. It is rapidly absorbed and easily digested.

To obtain hemp oil for use as a food, hemp seeds are cold pressed in an oxygen free environment. It should then be bottled in a light-proof container, flushed with nitrogen and refrigerated to protect the delicate oils from oxidization. This will ensure that your oil is as fresh as can possibly be.

Hemp Oil has the amazing properties listed below:

Is one of the lowest in saturated fats, only eight percent of total oil volume.

Has the highest level of Essential Fatty Acids of any plant. Contains Gamma Linolenic acid, a rare oil that is highly beneficial for human growth and development.

Is best taken internally but you may also obtain the benefits from hemp seed oil by using it on your skin.

Has anti-aging properties and can be used with other oils, such as sweet almond and jojoba oils, to make excellent massage oil.

Australian law prohibits the sale of hemp products as a food. Current legislation is not only out dated, it has been held in place due to the lack of knowledge and fear that to legalize hemp foods would be sending out a mixed message and would create policing issues. That was six years ago. However, in late 2009, an application was again submitted and will be decided on in October 2011. Lets us hope that the politicians who make this decision are not afraid to help Australia become the last western country in the world to allow hemp as a food.

ORGANIC HEMP OIL - THE KING OF OILS

Hemp is a plant that is a major source of confusion for many. While it's true that some species of hemp are illegal due to the substance THC, which is a psychoactive molecule, not all of the species of Hemp contain THC.

Hemp oil gained prominence with the health conscious of the world in the 1990s. For years people used the oil until it was removed from the market because oil is made from the seeds of the cannabis plant. The DEA tried to say that the oil was illegal, but in HIA vs. DEA it was determined that hemp based food products, including Hemp oil were exempt from the Controlled Substances Act.

Today, Hemp oil returns to it's seat at the top of the world of nutrition and the cosmetic world. It is important to note that there are a couple different types of Hemp oil. There is an expeller pressed variety, which is a food type product. It is used in food and cosmetics. There is also a steam distilled essential oil made from the hemp plant which is also used in cosmetics and aromatherapy practices. Here we are talking about the expeller pressed food product.

Use of the Hemp plant began in China sometime around 2300B.C. According to Chinese beliefs, the plant contains the prescription for immortality. The Chinese also used hemp oil to treat Malaria, menstrual problems and fertility.

In the 10th century, the Indians began to use the oil to treat indigestion, and anorexia as well as external wounds and infections, asthma, menstrual pain and more.

Until the beginning of this century, the plant fiber was used to make cloth, sails and ropes. However, in the interest of being environmentally friendly, many companies are once again producing fabric from Hemp fibers.

Hemp oil is rich with unsaturated fats and essential fatty acids. About 30-35% of the weight of the hemp seeds is the oil, which is pressed out in the production of the oil. The oil contains the essential fatty acids OMEGA 3 and OMEGA 6 at an optimal high rate, just like breast milk. The oil also contains protein, essential vitamins and minerals, which makes it an ideal dietary supplement.

Essential fatty acids are the cornerstones of proper nutrition rehabilitation and healing the body from disease. Even in the cosmetics industry, Hemp oil leads the way. Clinical studies have shown that Hemp oil is particularly effective in healing severe skin problem such as atopic dermatitis all the way up to burns.

Hemp oil strengthens the immune system, helps maintain a healthy cardiovascular system, and is effective in helping the body fight a long list of conditions such as lowering "bad" cholesterol, raising "good" cholesterol, lowering blood pressure and reducing the risk of heart attack, as well as being anti-inflammatory.

If you are a cancer sufferer and are undergoing chemotherapy, using Hemp oil is recommended at the same time. It encourages healthy cell creation and reduces the damage to the body as a result of treatment. The oil doesn't conflict with traditional medicinal treatments and is not a cure, but rather is complimentary.

BRIEF HISTORY OF CBD AND HEMP OIL

Cannabidiol (CBD) has been enjoying increasing amounts of attention as people learn more about its incredible possibilities as a supplement. With so many articles and research studies being written about CBD, you might think that this consumable is a recent discovery. It is true that many of the CBD extraction and packaging methods use cutting-edge technologies but the use of CBD in its hemp oil form goes back farther than most people realize.

In the 2010's the public began to see what a profound effect CBD oil could have treating a variety of life threatening aliments, especially in children. A prime example of this is a young family from Missoula Montana, using CBD oil to treat their 20 month old son, Cash Hyde, who had been diagnosed with brain cancer in 2010. Hyde's condition was worsening and his tumor inoperable. After exhausting every treatment option, including 30 rounds of intensive radiation, Ketamine, Methadone and Morphine treatments, the Hyde family had hit their limit. Nothing had worked. In an effort to give his small child some relief, his father did what was thought to be "crazy"at the time, and gave him a highly concentrated cannabis extract, not knowing what else to do. After the first treatment, Hyde's State IV brain tumor had shrunk. Although it was considered unorthodox, Mike Hyde was applauded by medical professionals and even spoke with the press in hopes of shedding the light on how CBD oil is literally a lifesaver. Cash Hyde lived for another two and a half years, passing away after the State of Montana made a change in legislation that impaired the family from easily accessing the cannabis oil their son needed.

Perhaps the most prolific case of CBD oil and it's success is the 2013 story that achieved national press. Charolette Figi is a 3 year old Colorado girl who suffered 300 grand mal seizures every week. Like the Hyde family, her parents thought they had tried everything, including a heavy regime of pharmaceutical drugs and painful procedures that still did not ease her condition. Her parents had watched a documentary of one of the first medical marijuana dispensaries in California centered around testing their strains of CBD and other cannaboid content. The California center testing was one of the first public assertions that cannabis was safe to ingest and use for a variety of medical purposes. CBD rich oil was able to treat 99% of the young girls seizures, and CNN aired a 2013 special on marijuana and it medicinal effects.

These are just a few specific instances that show how effective CBD oil can be, laying the groundwork for CBD oil being recognized as a justifiable medicine for a variety of ailments. As a result, many states are passing legislation rapidly allowing CBD oil to be used in numerous clinical studies as treatment plans. Research continues to back up it legitimacy and programs are being funded globally to continue the studies

ORGANIC HEMP OIL - THE KING OF OILS

Hemp is a plant that is a major source of confusion for many. While it's true that some species of hemp are illegal due to the substance THC, which is a psychoactive molecule, not all of the species of Hemp contain THC.

Hemp oil gained prominence with the health conscious of the world in the 1990s. For years people used the oil until it was removed from the market because oil is made from the seeds of the cannabis plant. The DEA tried to say that the oil was illegal, but in HIA vs. DEA it was determined that hemp based food products, including Hemp oil were exempt from the Controlled Substances Act.

Today, Hemp oil returns to its seat at the top of the world of nutrition and the cosmetic world. It is important to note that there are a couple different types of Hemp oil. There is an expeller pressed variety, which is a food type product. It is used in food and cosmetics. There is also a steam distilled essential oil made from the hemp plant which is also used in cosmetics and aromatherapy practices. Here we are talking about the expeller pressed food product.

Use of the Hemp plant began in China sometime around 2300B.C. According to Chinese beliefs, the plant contains the prescription for immortality. The Chinese also used hemp oil to treat Malaria, menstrual problems and fertility.

In the 10th century, the Indians began to use the oil to treat indigestion, and anorexia as well as external wounds and infections, asthma, menstrual pain and more.

Until the beginning of this century, the plant fiber was used to make cloth, sails and ropes. However, in the interest of being environmentally friendly, many companies are once again producing fabric from Hemp fibers.

Hemp oil is rich with unsaturated fats and essential fatty acids. About 30-35% of the weight of the hemp seeds is the oil, which is pressed out in the production of the oil. The oil contains the essential fatty acids OMEGA 3 and OMEGA 6 at an optimal high rate, just like breast milk. The oil also contains protein, essential vitamins and minerals, which makes it an ideal dietary supplement.

Essential fatty acids are the cornerstones of proper nutrition rehabilitation and healing the body from disease. Even in the cosmetics industry, Hemp oil leads the way. Clinical studies have shown that Hemp oil is particularly effective in healing severe skin problem such as atopic dermatitis all the way up to burns.

Hemp oil strengthens the immune system, helps maintain a healthy cardiovascular system, and is effective in helping the body fight a long list of conditions such as lowering "bad" cholesterol, raising "good" cholesterol, lowering blood pressure and reducing the risk of heart attack, as well as being anti-inflammatory.

If you are a cancer sufferer and are undergoing chemotherapy, using Hemp oil is recommended at the same time. It encourages healthy cell creation and reduces the damage to the body as a result of treatment. The oil doesn't conflict with traditional medicinal treatments and is not a cure, but rather is complimentary.

CBD HEMP OIL HEALTH BENEFITS: WHAT IS CBD HEMP OIL?

"Take Control of Your Health Naturally"
What is CBD Hemp Oil?
CBD, also called Cannabidiol, is just one of 85 different chemical compounds in marijuana plants. CBD Hemp Oil is derived from hemp, or cannabis grown with very little THC (often less than 0.3%). For the sake of this article we will refer to marijuana as cannabis grown for its psychoactive effects, and hemp as cannabis grown for its practical uses as a fiber. Marijuana is marketed for its THC content and hemp is utilized for its CBD content.
THC is the psychoactive or intoxicating compound found in cannabis plants whereas, CBD oil is not psychoactive or intoxicating and has shown strong signs of being an effective treatment for a variety of diseases and mental health disorders.

Where Can I Get CBD Hemp Oil?
Hemp oil is legal in all 50 states but the production of CBD Hemp Oil is not. Even though both come from marijuana, hemp oil is derived from sterile cannabis seeds, which are legal under the Controlled Substances Act. CBD Oil is derived from the plant's flowers which are not legal in some states. However, this doesn't stop the import of CBD oil made from industrialized hemp grown legally, which is why you're able to buy it legally on the internet.

You can find products containing hemp oil in the beauty section of your local retail store, but to get CBD Oil you'll either need to be in a state where it's legal to produce or purchase an import.

CBD Hemp Oil Health Benefits

CBD Oil has been shown to have surprisingly positive effects on a variety of diseases. Some of the Cannabidiol health benefits are:

> - Nausea treatment
> - Lowered anxiety
> - Pain relief
> - Improved mood
> - Lessening withdrawal symptoms
> - Seizure reduction
> - Stimulating appetite

CBD works by activating the body's serotonin (anti-depressant effect), vanilloid (pain relief), and adenosine (anti-inflammatory effect) receptors. How quickly you start to feel the results from CBD Oil depends on how it was ingested and your weight. Someone small who ingested the oil in spray form will feel the effects much faster than a larger person ingesting CBD in capsule form.

Different Forms of CBD Hemp Oil

CBD Hemp Oil can take on many different forms, including liquids, ointments, and sprays, and capsules. Most oils and sprays are used by putting the substance under your tongue. Ointments are used on and absorbed by the skin, and thirdly capsules are ingested. Those who don't like the taste of sprays or oils can defer to capsules. Capsules are a very convenient way to consume Cannabidiol, however you don't absorb as much CBD from a capsule as you do from an oil or spray put under your tongue.

CBD vape oil is the same as regular CBD Hemp Oil - it's just taken into the body in a different way. You just fill your vape pen with Cannabidiol and presto, you've got yourself a vape with health benefits.

CBD Oil sold online are not as potent as those medically prescribed for serious diseases but they can help with mood disorders, lower anxiety, and lessen pain caused by inflammation.

CBD Hemp Oil Side Effects

While not much research has been done yet on the side effects of CBD Oil, whether absorbed, swallowed as a capsule or inhaled through a CBD vape pen, the most commonly side effects reported are digestive issues, such as upset stomach and diarrhea, which are not very common.

Will CBD Hemp oil Show on a Drug Test?

Drug tests are looking for THC, not CBD, and because CBD doesn't produce any kind of high, employers really have no reason to look for it in the first place. So CBD Oil does not show up on a drug test. However, for this reason, make sure you purchase pure CBD oil with 0% THC.

Unique Benefits of Using Pure CBD Oil

No prescription required: Even though they are more potent than regular CBD Oils, most pure CBD Oils do not require a prescription.

0% THC: If you're worried about using a cannabis extract because you don't want to experience marijuana's psychoactive effects or fail a drug test, opt for pure CBD Oil. Containing no THC at all, it's the safest choice.

Fewer side effects: Pure CBD Oils are less likely to cause nausea and fatigue.

Purchase Cautions: How do you know if you are getting quality CBD Hemp Oil?

Your first clue is usually price. If the price seems too cheap to be true, it probably is.

Always purchase from a reputable source. A company that is reputable will back their product and will not risk selling misrepresented items.

Another thing to look for is the way that the product is marketed. If you see CBD Hemp Oil online that claims to cure every ailment under the sun, it's also probably too good to be true.

The top products are made from organically grown hemp and have a CBD concentration over 20mg.

While the medicinal effects of Cannabidiol are great, keep your expectations of online brands realistic.

HOW TO USE THE CBD HEMP OIL

CBD oil is used in different ways to relieve the symptoms of different conditions.

Some CBD oil products can be mixed into different foods or drinks, taken from a pipette or dropper, or are available as a thick paste to be massaged into the skin. CBD can also be purchased in capsule form.

Other products are provided as sprays that are meant to be administered under the tongue.

Here are a few recommended dosages, although these may vary between individuals based on other factors, such as body weight, the concentration of the product, and the condition being treated.

Due to the lack of FDA regulation for CBD products, seek advice from a medical professional before settling on any particular dosage.

All dosages relate to taking CBD oil by mouth. These can include:
Chronic pain: Take between 2.5 and 20 milligrams (mg) by mouth for no more than 25 days.
Epilepsy: Consume between 200 and 300 mg of CBD by mouth daily for up to 4.5 months.
Movement problems associated with Huntington's disease: Taking 10 mg every day for six weeks can help ease movements.
Sleep disorders: Take between 40 and 160 mg.
Schizophrenia: Consume between 40 and 1,280 mg CBD by mouth daily for up to 4 weeks.
Glaucoma: One dose of between 20 and 40 mg applied under the tongue can help to relieve pressure in the eye. However, caution is advised - doses greater than 40 mg might actually increase pressure.
As regulation in the U.S. increases, more exact doses and prescriptions will start to emerge.
After discussing dosage and risks with a doctor, and researching regional legal use, it is important to compare different brands. There are a range of different CBD oils available to purchase online, with different benefits and applications.

HEMP OIL, HEMP PROTEIN - EXCELLENT HELP IN SUPPRESSING APPETITE

Hemp. Some people use its fibrous stalks to make ropes. And admittedly, looking to a plant from which ropes are made might seem like a strange place to look for something that can help dieters succeed in their weight-loss efforts. But amazingly, the hemp plant provides just that. Hemp seeds are filled with oil, and cold-pressed hemp oil is in fact one of the most nutritionally dense foods on the planet, and as a bonus, helps with suppressing appetite.

Hemp comes in various forms suitable for dietary consumption. For example, the seeds can be eaten raw, ground into a meal called hemp protein, sprouted, turned into hemp milk (similar to soymilk), or used as a tea.

Similar in many ways to flax seed, hemp seed contains high amounts of protein, and its oil is rich in omega 3 essential fatty acids (EFAs). In fact, hemp contains about 20 percent highly digestible protein, and omega 3 EFAs make up about 22 percent of its oil.

It's the omega 3s that give hemp its ability to suppress appetite. Recent research reported in the journal Appetite showed that study volunteers who ate a dinner rich in omega 3s were significantly less hungry, both afterward and even two hours later, than those whose dinners contained no omega 3s but were otherwise virtually identical. Omega 3 oils, it turns out, somehow help regulate the brain's hunger signal center.

Other research has shown that hemp's benefits extend beyond appetite suppression. Research has also shown hemp to help relieve symptoms of eczema, and its omega 3s are known to help improve memory and brain function.

When you're doing your level best to lose weight, finding natural ways to subdue your appetite gives you a definite edge in your efforts. And one of the best, proven items to add to your appetite-suppression arsenal is hemp...its seeds, oil, and protein.

I'm Ken McFarland, and if you'd like to learn more, I invite you to visit [http://www.natural-appetitesuppressants.com], where you can learn about a wide variety of foods that can help you stop being hungry [http://www.natural-appetitesuppressants.com] so much and therefore make it ever so much easier to lose weight.

HEMP OIL BENEFITS THAT PEOPLE OUGHT TO KNOW

Many people are very fond of using beauty products like body oils and lotions that are manufactured by leading companies. But because these products are quite expensive, not all people are able to enjoy them. But the good news for other people who want to try skin care products is that there are alternatives that even provide better benefits. Hemp oil's benefits compared to other products are better and more effective in achieving optimum health condition.

Hemp oil is produced after pressing hemp seeds. This oil is known to be rich in several nutrients needed by the body; some of these are the Omega 6 and Omega 3, amino acids, and other essential fatty acids. According to World Health Organization (WHO), these acids are needed by the body for optimal health.

Although the oil is believed to provide a lot of benefits, other people are still hesitant about it. Because it contains tetrahydrocannabinol, people think it is not as healthy as it appears. But according to companies that manufacture hemp oil, only the seed contains this element; therefore, these elements are removed during the process of pressing the seeds to extract the oil.

In other countries, hemp seeds are not used to produce food, and are not recommended for human consumption. However, they can be used to produce skin care or industrial products. For skin care products made of hemp seeds, there are many positive benefits that can be expected.

Hemp oil has several properties that make it one of the best products when it comes to skin care:

Gentle for anyone.

People have different skin types, which is why it's very important to use a product that won't trigger allergic reactions. Hemp oil is ideal for different types of skin.

It's an anti-inflammatory product.

People suffering from skin irritation, redness, rashes and other skin issues can safely use the oil as it alleviates these symptoms. Also, people who have eczema, acne, psoriasis, and dermatitis can safely use this oil. It's very safe for the skin.

It contains moisturizers.

Hemp oil contains essential fatty acids, which make it effective to act as a moisturizer. This could very well help people who have oily and dry skin. Unlike the greasy feeling brought by other body oils or lotions, hemp oil makes the skin moisturized all day without getting the pores clogged.

· It's perfect for hair care.
A lot of conditioners and shampoos today contain hemp oil. Since it contains a good amount of conditioning nutrients, it's perfect for making the hair stronger and thicker.
Besides skin care benefits, the oil can also be used to reduce swelling and pain caused by osteoporosis and arthritis. Furthermore, it helps in relieving premenstrual stress, absorbing calcium, and acts as an ordinary sunblock.

HEMP OIL: A SUPER FOOD

For all of you who are still on the "Just Say No" bandwagon, you might believe that hemp seed oil, which is derived from the seeds of the cannabis plant, is just another way for those dang hippies to get high. However, while the flowers this controversial plant are capable of bringing about mild hallucinations and making everything on FOX News seem hilarious, the seeds and the beneficial fatty oils that they contain, will do no such thing. In fact, hemp seed oil is thought to be one of the most beneficial supplements a person can take in order to maintain an active and healthy lifestyle.

Once upon a time before politicians and business interests got involved, hemp was an important crop with any industrial and medicinal uses. On the health front, the seeds of the hemp plant were found to be an almost perfect food source, containing 80% of the essential fatty acids that our bodies need as well as globule edestins which is a rare protein that is similar to globulin. Hemp oil is easily digestible and contains pretty much all of the essential fatty acids that the body needs in order to stay functioning properly. Modern Research studies have found that taking hemp oil on a regular basis can help repair a damaged immune system and even reverse wasting making it an important natural supplement for both cancer patients and people with AIDS

Taking Internally Hemp Oil Can:
Increase vitality
Help with motor skills
Ease Arthritis Pain
Strengthen the Immune System
Treat Tuberculosis
Decrease Sun Related Damage to the skin
People with conditions caused by deficiency in LA (Omega 6) and LNA (Omega 3) can be treated by taking hemp oil because it has those essential fatty acids (EFA) in balanced, ideal proportions.

Hemp seed oil has a low level of Stearic acid (18:0) which is beneficial for health because high levels of Stearic acid form flow-impeding clots in blood vessels and work against the healing qualities of the EFA's.

How much to take:

On the daily basis you can take 2-4 dessert spoons (up to 50 ml) per day. In the case of therapy you can increase the dose up to 150 ml per day for approximately 7 days, then return to the regular daily amount.

Hemp Seed Oil has a nutty flavor that most people find pleasant. It is an ideal additive to salad dressings, dips, or cold pasta. It is not suitable for frying, since excess heat will greatly reduce many of its life giving benefits. It can also be used externally to treat skin conditions such as eczema. You can find it many health food stores.

HEMP OIL IS ONE OF THE FEW OILS THAT IS RICH IN ESSENTIAL FATTY ACIDS (EFAS) OMEGA-3, OMEGA-6, & 9

Hemp oil is one of the few oils that is rich in Essential Fatty Acids (EFAs). Essential Fatty Acids are fats that the body requires for healthy cells but cannot manufacture by itself. EFAs include Polyunsaturated Fatty Acids (PUFAs), Omega-3, Omega-6, Omega-9, Linoleic Acid and Gamma Linolenic Acid (GLA).

Although it is very important in skin care and maintenance, GLAs are rarely found in natural oils. Some excellent sources are from the seeds of evening primrose, borage and hemp.

Research

In cosmetic testing, EFAs have been shown to play a preventive role in the skin aging process. The outflow of moisture from the body is regulated by a barrier which the skin forms to protect itself from the external environment. EFAs, particularly Omega-6 and GLA, preserve the "barrier function" of cell membranes. Skin which is deficient in these nutrients allows more moisture loss and can show dryness and loss of elasticity. PUFAs have also been shown to prevent skin dryness and to help restore damaged skin to normal. Omega 6 and Omega 3 EFA's are required more in our diet than any other vitamin, and yet our bodies do not produce them naturally. These oils must be ingested in their pure form, as they can not be metabolized from other food sources. These healing enzymes can be absorbed directly into the skin to replenish missing oils, so they are ideally suited for many cosmetics and skin care products.

Hemp oil also provides an ample supply of carotene, phytosterols, and phospholipids, in addition to a large number of minerals including: calcium, sulfur, magnesium, phosphorus and potassium. It is also a good source of chlorophyll.

Due to its rich content of Essential Fatty Acids, hemp seed oil is a perfect choice for skin, hair & lip care.

Hemp Oil Naturally Replenishes Skin Moisture!

Hemp Oil is the only oil of its kind that helps soothe skin irritation and dryness! If you suffer from:

- ➢ **Eczema**
- ➢ **Psoriasis**
- ➢ **Skin cracking, scaling or sagging**
- ➢ **Chapped lips**
- ➢ **Dry hair**
- ➢ **Substantially improve your skin's natural appearance and elasticity**

When combined with other naturally derived ingredients such as carrier oils, herbs and essential oils, it offers an exceptional solution to many skin types and conditons. In addition, hemp helps to preserve eco-systems that are subject to toxic chemically laden products on a daily basis.

Everyone can truly benefit from this versatile plant. Continuous use of skin-care products containing Omega-6 fatty acids can restore your skin's natural glow and bring a healthy sheen to your hair and lips. Because hemp oil is an excellent source of Omega fatty acids, adding it to your diet can substantially improve your skin's natural appearance and elasticity. The result is healthy, moisturized and silky smooth skin! Who knew cooking oil could do all that!

MORE ABOUT CBD HEMP OIL

What is CBD oil?

CBD is one of many compounds, known as cannabinoids, that are found in the cannabis plant. Researchers have been looking at the potential therapeutic uses of CBD.

Oils that contain concentrations of CBD are known as CBD oils. The concentration and uses of different oils vary.

Cannabidiol oil is used for health purposes, but it is controversial. There is some confusion about what it is and the effect it has on the human body.

Cannabidiol (CBD) may have some health benefits, but there may also be some risks. It is also not legal in every state.

Is CBD marijuana?

CBD oil is a cannabinoid derived from the cannabis plant. Until recently, the most well-known compound in cannabis was delta-9 tetrahydrocannabinol (THC). This is the most active ingredient in marijuana.

Marijuana contains both THC and CBD, but the compounds have different effects. THC is well-known for the mind-altering "high" it produces when broken down by heat and introduced into the body, such as when smoking the plant or cooking it into foods.

'

Unlike THC, CBD is not psychoactive. This means that it does not change the state of mind of the person who uses it. However, it does appear to produce significant changes in the body and has been found to have medical benefits.

Most of the CBD used medicinally is found in the least processed form of the cannabis plant, known as hemp.

Hemp and marijuana come from the same plant, cannabis sativa, but they are very different.

Over the years, marijuana farmers have selectively bred their plants to be very high in THC and other compounds that interested them, either for a smell or an effect they had on the plant's flowers.

On the other hand, hemp farmers have not tended to modify the plant. It is these hemp plants that are used to create CBD oil.

How CBD works

All cannabinoids, including CBD, attach themselves to certain receptors in the body to produce their effects.

The human body produces certain cannabinoids on its own. It has two receptors for cannabinoids, called CB1 receptors and CB2 receptors.

CB1 receptors are found all around the body, but many of them are in the brain.

The CB1 receptors in the brain deal with coordination and movement, pain, emotions and mood, thinking, appetite, and memories, among others. THC attaches to these receptors.

CB2 receptors are more common in the immune system. They affect inflammation and pain.

It used to be thought that CBD acts on these CB2 receptors, but it appears now that CBD does not act on either receptor directly. Instead, it seems to influence the body to use more of its own cannabinoids.

LEGALITY

Cannabis is legal for either medicinal or recreational use in some but not all states. Other states approve CBD oil as a hemp product without approving the general use of medical marijuana.

Laws may differ between federal and state level, and current marijuana and CBD legislation in the United States can be confusing, even in states where marijuana is legal.

There is an ever-changing number of states that do not necessarily consider marijuana to be legal but have laws directly related to CBD oil. This information is up to date as of July 24, 2017, but the laws frequently change.

The laws vary, but they generally approve CBD oil as legal for treating a range of epileptic conditions at various concentrations. A full list of states that have CBD-specific laws is available here.

Different states also require different levels of prescription to possess and use CBD oil. In Missouri, for example, a person must show that three other treatment options have been unsuccessful in treating epilepsy.

If you are considering CBD oil as a treatment for a suitable condition, talk to your local healthcare provider. They will have an understanding of safe CBD sources and local laws surrounding usage. Research the laws for your own state. In most cases, a prescription will be required.

CBD SIDE EFFECTS AND RISK

Many small-scale studies have looked into the safety of CBD in adults and found that it is well tolerated across a wide range of doses.

There have been no significant side effects in the central nervous system or effects on vital signs and mood among people who use it either slightly or heavily.

The most common side effect noted is tiredness. Some people have noticed diarrhea and changes in appetite or weight.

There are still very little long-term safety data available, and, to date, tests have not been carried out on children.

As with any new or alternative treatment option, a patient should discuss CBD with a qualified healthcare practitioner before use.

The United States Food and Drug Administration (FDA) has not approved CBD for the treatment of any condition. It can be difficult to know whether a product contains a safe or effective level of CBD or whether the product has the properties and contents stated on its packaging and marketing.

OTHER SIDE EFFECTS ARE:

Though CBD is generally well tolerated and considered safe, it may cause adverse reactions in some people.
Side effects noted in studies include
- ➢ **Anxiety and depression**
- ➢ **Psychosis**
- ➢ **Nausea**
- ➢ **Vomiting**
- ➢ **Drowsiness**
- ➢ **Dry mouth**
- ➢ **Dizziness**
- ➢ **Diarrhea**
- ➢ **Changes in appetite**

CBD is also known to interact with several medications. Before you start using CBD oil, discuss it with your doctor to ensure your safety and avoid potentially harmful interactions